Pocket Atlas
of Normal CT Anatomy

James B. Weinstein, M.D.
Instructor in Radiology
(Currently at Northside Radiology Associates, P.A.,
Atlanta, Georgia)

Joseph K. T. Lee, M.D.
Associate Professor of Radiology
Co-Director, Computed Body Tomography Section

Stuart S. Sagel, M.D.
Professor of Radiology
Director, Chest Radiology Section
Co-Director, Computed Body Tomography Section

Mallinckrodt Institute of Radiology
Washington University School of Medicine
St. Louis, Missouri

Raven Press   New York

Raven Press, 1185 Avenue of the Americas, New York, New York 10036

© 1985 by Raven Press Books, Ltd. All rights reserved. This book is protected
by copyright. No part of it may be reproduced, stored in a retrieval system, or
transmitted, in any form or by any means, electronic, mechanical, photocopying,
recording, or otherwise, without the prior written permission of the publisher.

Made in the United States of America

Library of Congress Cataloging in Publication Data

Weinstein, James B.
  Pocket atlas of normal CT anatomy.

  1. Tomography—Atlases.   2. Anatomy, Human—Atlases.
I. Lee, Joseph K. T.   II. Sagel, Stuart S., 1940–
III. Title.   IV. Title: Pocket atlas of normal C.T.
anatomy.   [DNLM: 1. Anatomy—atlases.   2. Tomography,
X-Ray Computed—atlases.   QS 17 W424p]
RC78.7.T6W45   1985   616.07′572   84-42781
ISBN 0-88167-070-7

The material contained in this volume was submitted as previously unpublished
material, except in the instances in which credit has been given to the source from
which some of the illustrative material was derived.
  Great care has been taken to maintain the accuracy of the information contained
in the volume. However, Raven Press cannot be held responsible for errors or for
any consequences arising from the use of the information contained herein.

9 8 7 6 5 4 3

Preface

Since its inception, the study of computed tomography (CT) has relied on a thorough understanding of normal gross anatomy. Although several excellent and detailed texts on cross-sectional anatomy exist, a concise, pocket-sized atlas of body CT anatomy has been unavailable until now. This atlas contains high-quality, state-of-the-art CT images of the neck and larynx, chest, abdomen, and pelvis. CT scans and the accompanying line drawings appear on facing pages and are arranged from cephalad to caudad within each anatomic section. For simplicity, structures which appear in more than one scan may only be labeled once. Dashed lines in the drawings indicate bone or cartilage. The level of each CT scan is indicated by the horizontal lines on the drawing of the torso on the first page of each section. The number to the left of each line corresponds to the page number of the scan.

This work is intended for those learning basic CT anatomy including radiologists in practice and in training, physicians in the clinical specialties, and medical students. This atlas will serve as a convenient source of knowledge of anatomy as applied to CT.

fat   −50 to −100

This atlas is dedicated to Roy R. Peterson, Ph.D., Professor of Anatomy at Washington University, for his expertise, advice, and inspiration in the study of gross anatomy.

Acknowledgments

We would like to thank the following: our secretaries Sue Day, Patty Haring, Carol Keller, and Lynn Losse; Cramer Lewis and staff in the Department of Medical Illustration for photographic work; Vicki Friedman and Marci Hartstein for their skill in preparing the line drawings.

4

Contents

Neck and Larynx   6
Chest   20
Abdomen   38
Male Pelvis   60
Female Pelvis   80

Neck and Larynx

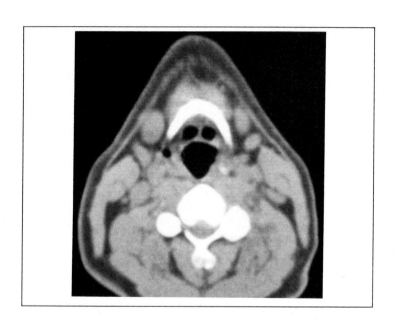

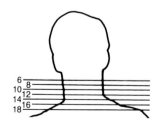

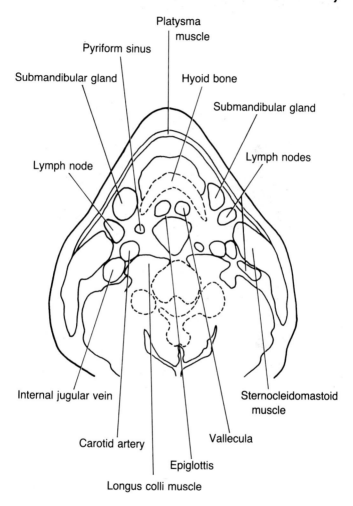

Platysma muscle

Pyriform sinus

Submandibular gland

Hyoid bone

Submandibular gland

Lymph node

Lymph nodes

Internal jugular vein

Sternocleidomastoid muscle

Carotid artery

Vallecula

Epiglottis

Longus colli muscle

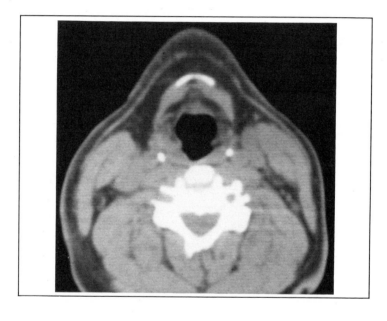

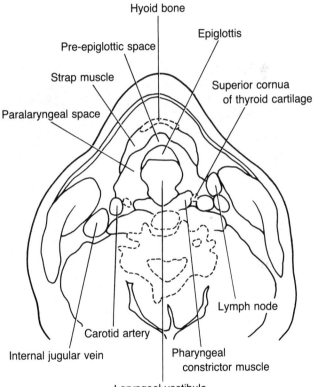

Hyoid bone

Epiglottis

Pre-epiglottic space

Strap muscle

Superior cornua
of thyroid cartilage

Paralaryngeal space

Lymph node

Carotid artery

Internal jugular vein

Pharyngeal
constrictor muscle

Laryngeal vestibule

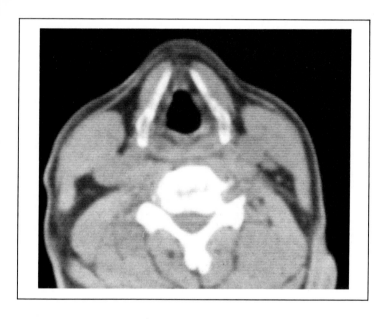

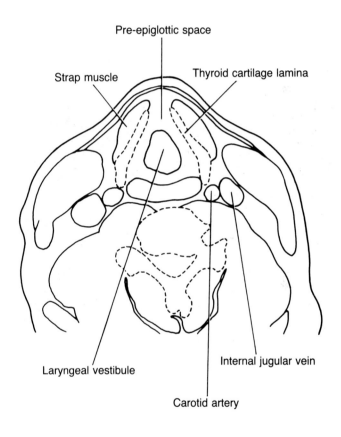

Pre-epiglottic space

Strap muscle

Thyroid cartilage lamina

Laryngeal vestibule

Internal jugular vein

Carotid artery

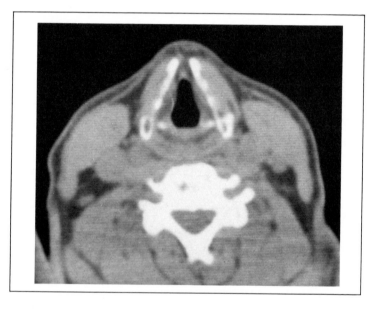

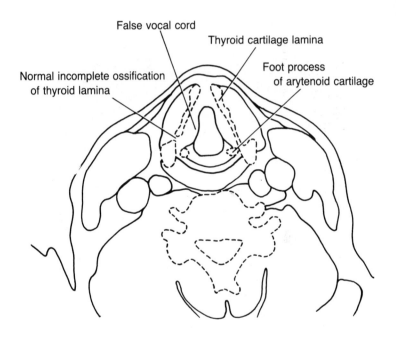

False vocal cord

Thyroid cartilage lamina

Foot process
of arytenoid cartilage

Normal incomplete ossification
of thyroid lamina

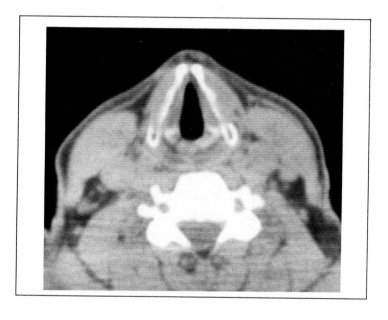

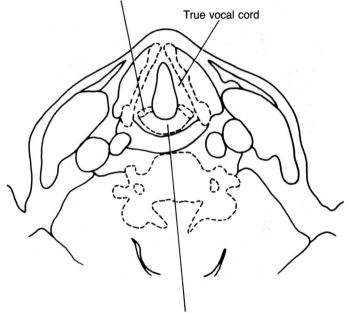

Vocal process of arytenoid cartilage

True vocal cord

Top of lamina of cricoid cartilage

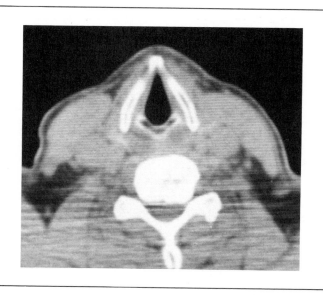

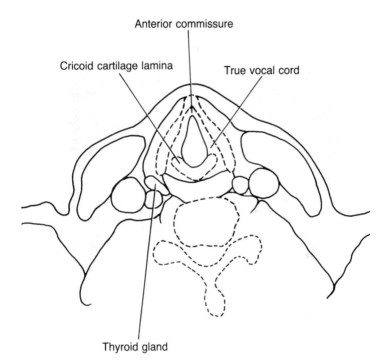

Anterior commissure

Cricoid cartilage lamina

True vocal cord

Thyroid gland

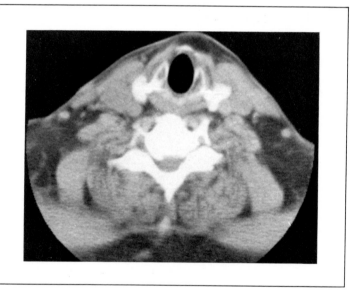

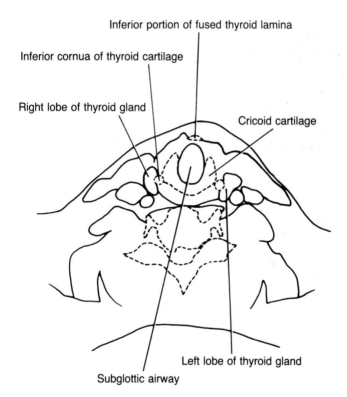

Inferior portion of fused thyroid lamina

Inferior cornua of thyroid cartilage

Right lobe of thyroid gland

Cricoid cartilage

Left lobe of thyroid gland

Subglottic airway

Chest

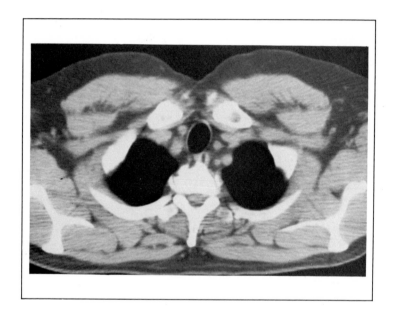

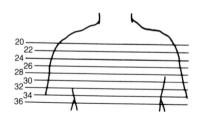

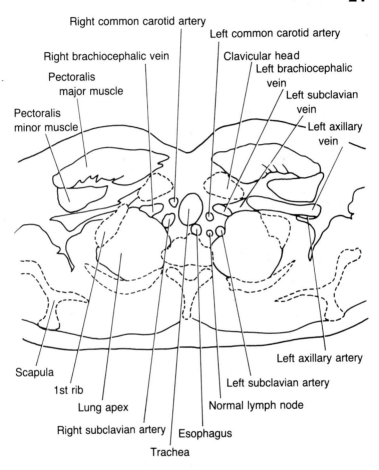

Right common carotid artery

Left common carotid artery

Right brachiocephalic vein

Clavicular head

Left brachiocephalic vein

Pectoralis major muscle

Left subclavian vein

Pectoralis minor muscle

Left axillary vein

Left axillary artery

Scapula

Left subclavian artery

1st rib

Normal lymph node

Lung apex

Right subclavian artery

Esophagus

Trachea

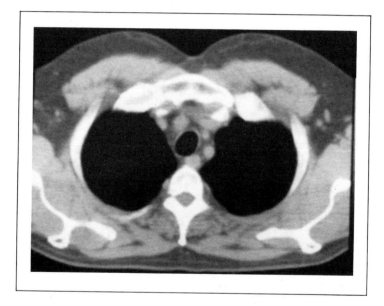

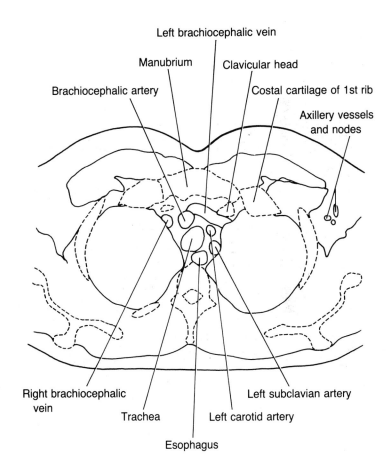

Left brachiocephalic vein

Manubrium

Clavicular head

Brachiocephalic artery

Costal cartilage of 1st rib

Axillery vessels
and nodes

Right brachiocephalic
vein

Left subclavian artery

Trachea

Left carotid artery

Esophagus

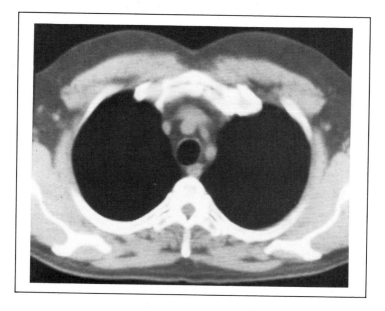

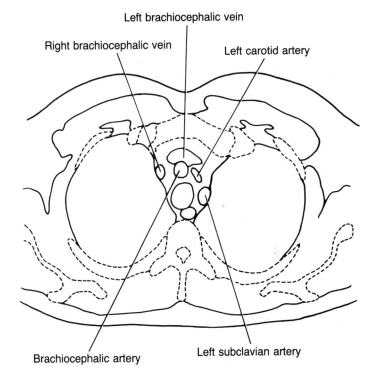

Left brachiocephalic vein

Right brachiocephalic vein

Left carotid artery

Brachiocephalic artery

Left subclavian artery

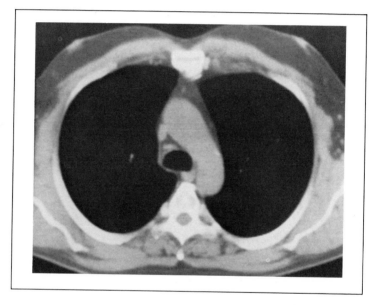

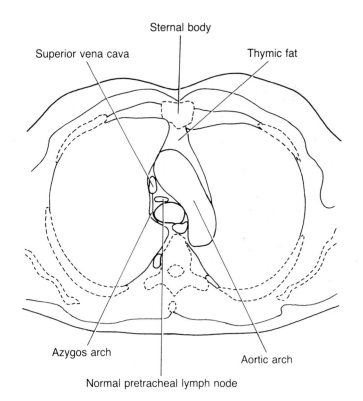

Sternal body

Superior vena cava

Thymic fat

Azygos arch

Aortic arch

Normal pretracheal lymph node

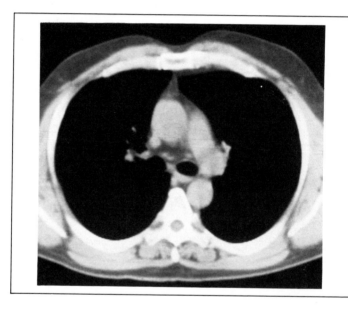

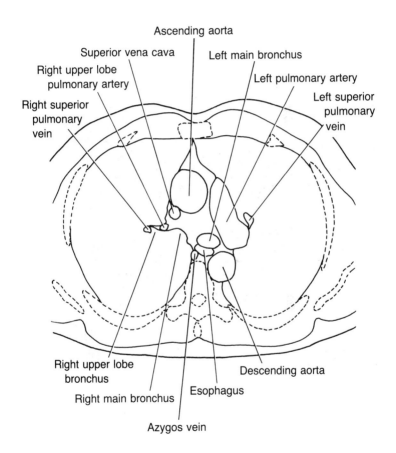

Ascending aorta

Superior vena cava

Left main bronchus

Right upper lobe
pulmonary artery

Left pulmonary artery

Right superior
pulmonary
vein

Left superior
pulmonary
vein

Right upper lobe
bronchus

Descending aorta

Right main bronchus

Esophagus

Azygos vein

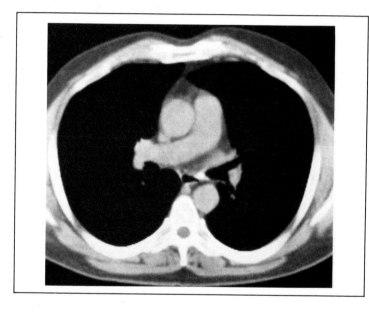

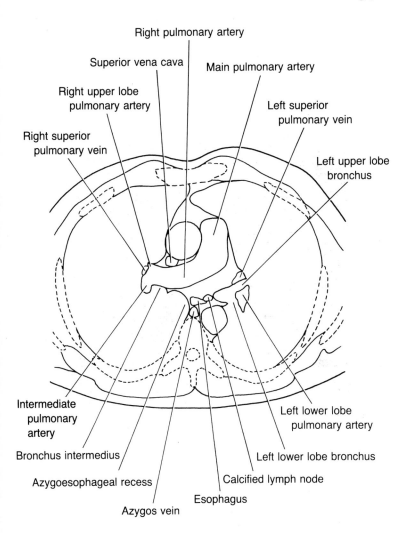

Right pulmonary artery

Superior vena cava

Main pulmonary artery

Right upper lobe
pulmonary artery

Left superior
pulmonary vein

Right superior
pulmonary vein

Left upper lobe
bronchus

Intermediate
pulmonary
artery

Left lower lobe
pulmonary artery

Bronchus intermedius

Left lower lobe bronchus

Azygoesophageal recess

Calcified lymph node

Azygos vein

Esophagus

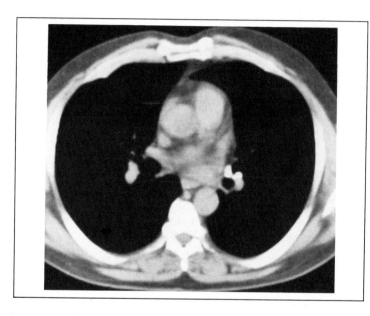

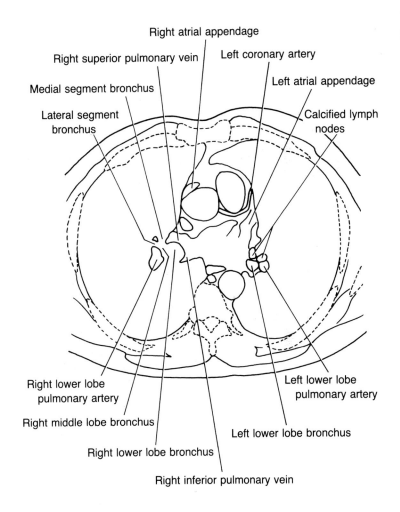

Right atrial appendage

Right superior pulmonary vein

Left coronary artery

Medial segment bronchus

Left atrial appendage

Lateral segment
bronchus

Calcified lymph
nodes

Right lower lobe
pulmonary artery

Left lower lobe
pulmonary artery

Right middle lobe bronchus

Left lower lobe bronchus

Right lower lobe bronchus

Right inferior pulmonary vein

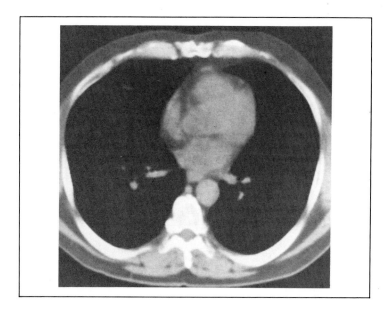

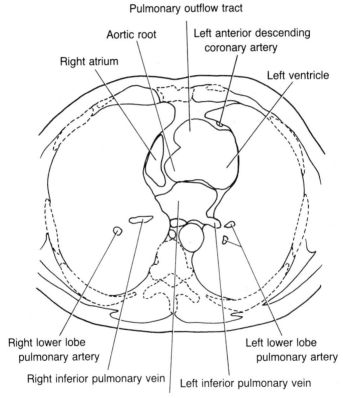

Pulmonary outflow tract

Aortic root

Left anterior descending coronary artery

Right atrium

Left ventricle

Right lower lobe pulmonary artery

Left lower lobe pulmonary artery

Right inferior pulmonary vein

Left inferior pulmonary vein

Left atrium

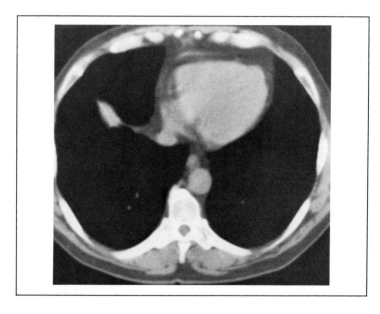

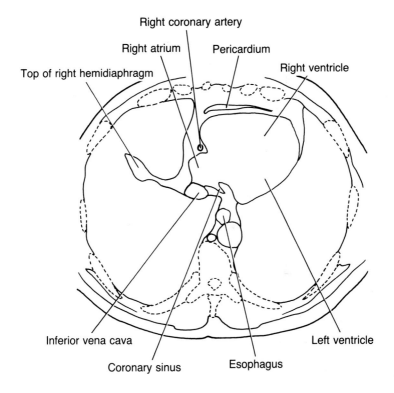

Right coronary artery

Right atrium   Pericardium

Top of right hemidiaphragm   Right ventricle

Inferior vena cava   Left ventricle

Coronary sinus   Esophagus

Abdomen

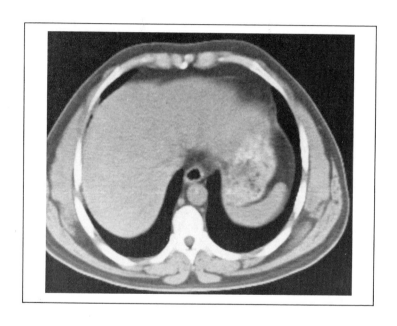

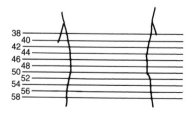

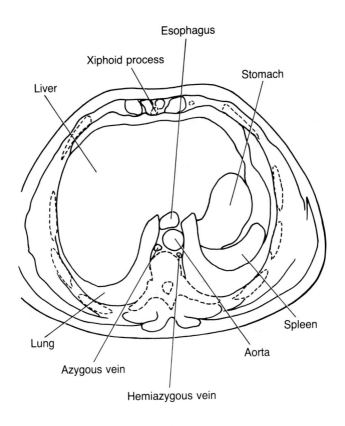

Esophagus

Xiphoid process

Stomach

Liver

Lung

Azygous vein

Hemiazygous vein

Aorta

Spleen

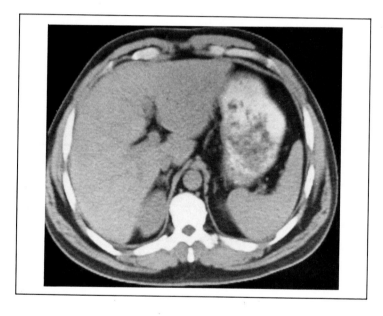

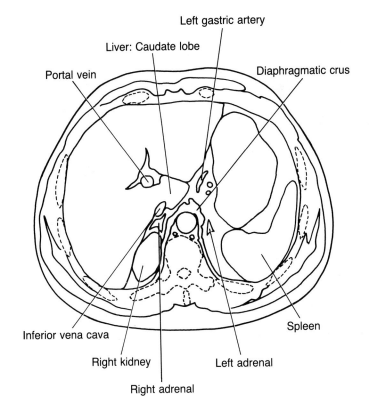

Left gastric artery

Liver: Caudate lobe

Portal vein

Diaphragmatic crus

Inferior vena cava

Spleen

Right kidney

Left adrenal

Right adrenal

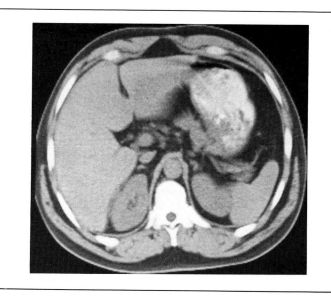

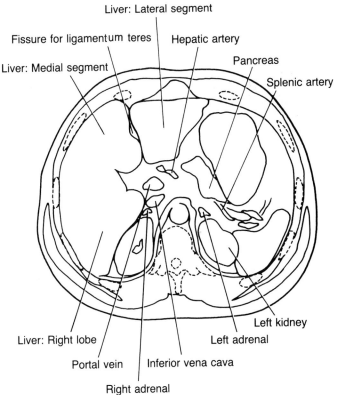

Liver: Lateral segment

Fissure for ligamentum teres

Hepatic artery

Liver: Medial segment

Pancreas

Splenic artery

Left kidney

Left adrenal

Liver: Right lobe

Inferior vena cava

Portal vein

Right adrenal

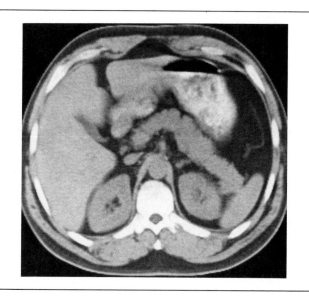

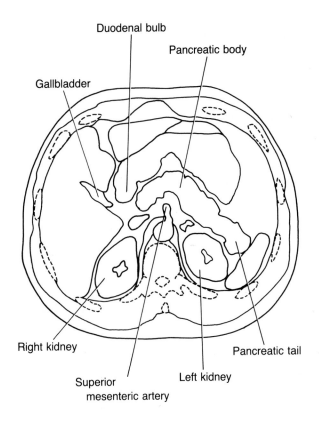

Duodenal bulb

Pancreatic body

Gallbladder

Right kidney

Superior
mesenteric artery

Left kidney

Pancreatic tail

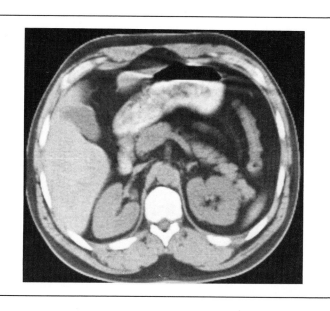

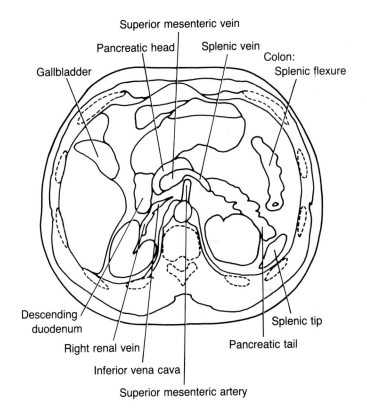

Superior mesenteric vein

Pancreatic head   Splenic vein

Gallbladder   Colon:
                                               Splenic flexure

Descending
duodenum   Splenic tip

Right renal vein   Pancreatic tail

Inferior vena cava

Superior mesenteric artery

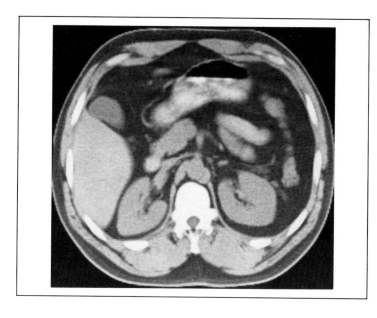

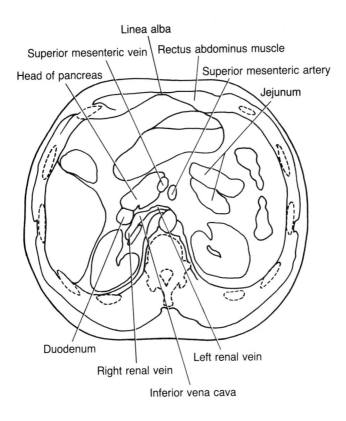

Linea alba

Superior mesenteric vein

Rectus abdominus muscle

Head of pancreas

Superior mesenteric artery

Jejunum

Duodenum

Left renal vein

Right renal vein

Inferior vena cava

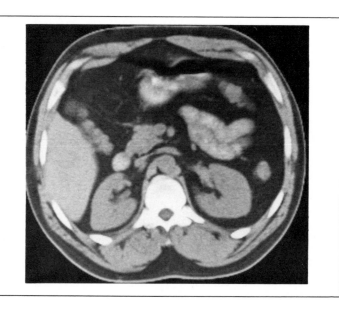

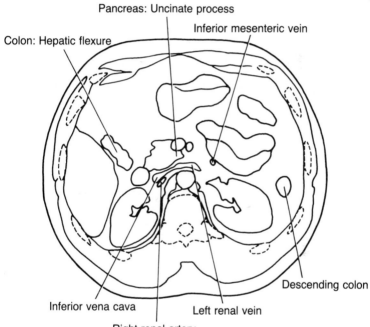

Pancreas: Uncinate process

Inferior mesenteric vein

Colon: Hepatic flexure

Inferior vena cava

Right renal artery

Left renal vein

Descending colon

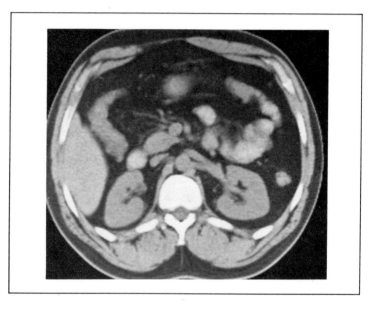

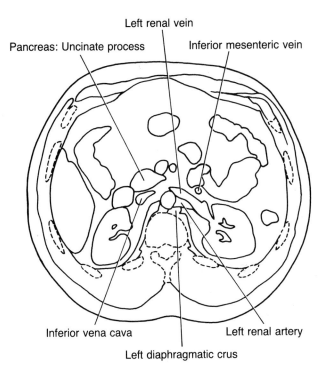

Left renal vein

Pancreas: Uncinate process

Inferior mesenteric vein

Inferior vena cava

Left renal artery

Left diaphragmatic crus

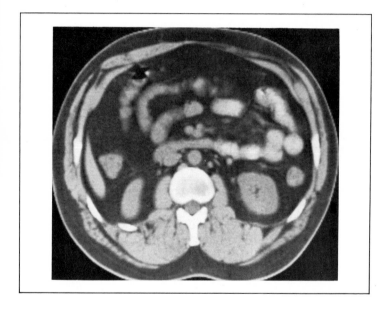

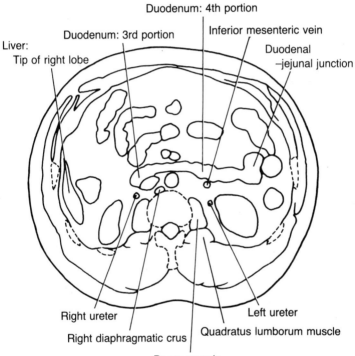

Duodenum: 4th portion

Inferior mesenteric vein

Duodenum: 3rd portion

Duodenal
–jejunal junction

Liver:
Tip of right lobe

Right ureter

Left ureter

Right diaphragmatic crus

Quadratus lumborum muscle

Psoas muscle

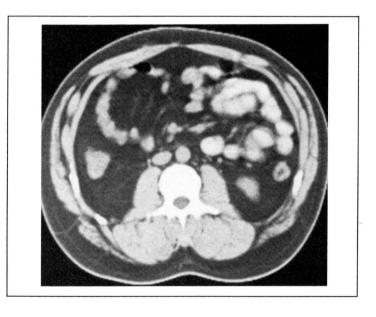

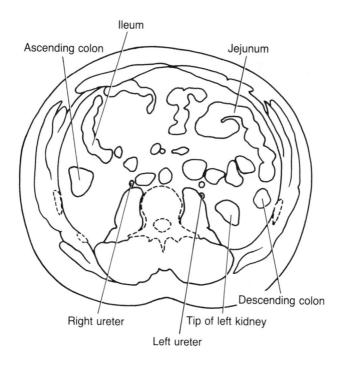

Ileum

Ascending colon

Jejunum

Right ureter

Tip of left kidney

Left ureter

Descending colon

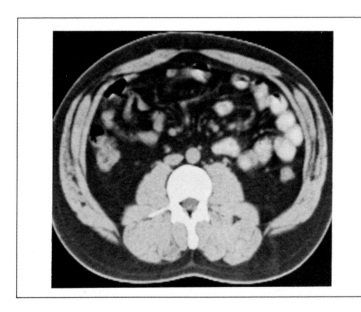

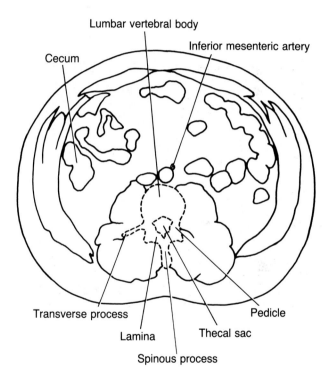

Lumbar vertebral body

Inferior mesenteric artery

Cecum

Transverse process

Lamina

Pedicle

Thecal sac

Spinous process

Male Pelvis

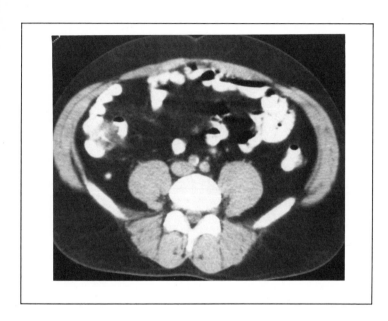

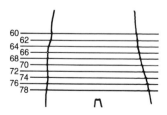

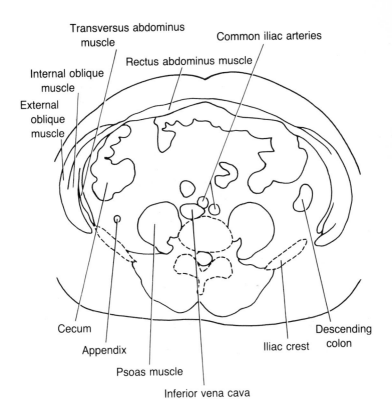

Transversus abdominus muscle

Common iliac arteries

Rectus abdominus muscle

Internal oblique muscle

External oblique muscle

Cecum

Appendix

Psoas muscle

Inferior vena cava

Iliac crest

Descending colon

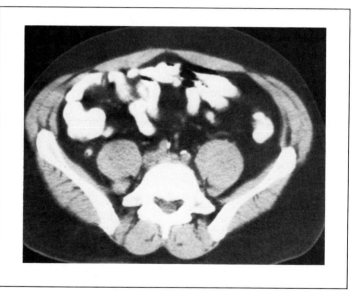

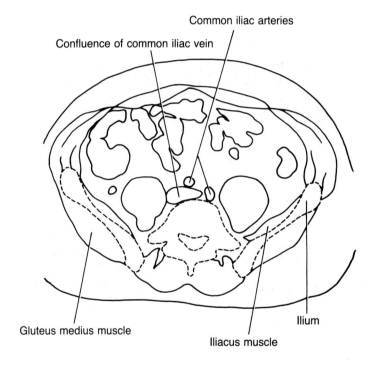

Common iliac arteries

Confluence of common iliac vein

Gluteus medius muscle

Iliacus muscle

Ilium

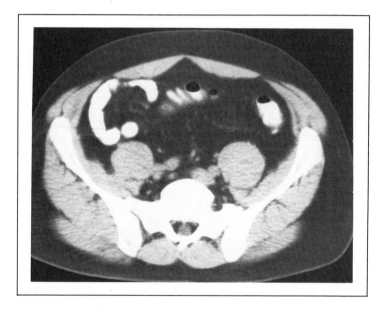

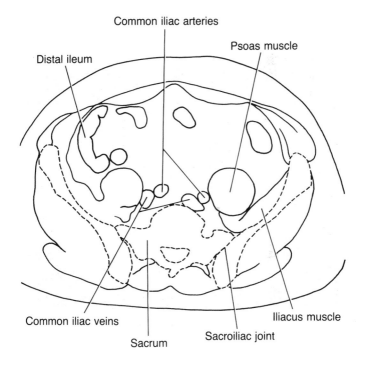

Common iliac arteries

Psoas muscle

Distal ileum

Common iliac veins

Sacrum

Sacroiliac joint

Iliacus muscle

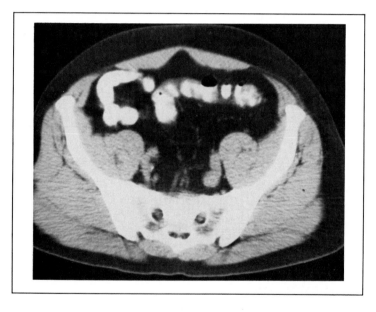

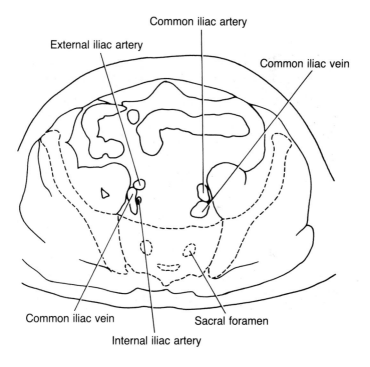

Common iliac artery

External iliac artery

Common iliac vein

Common iliac vein

Internal iliac artery

Sacral foramen

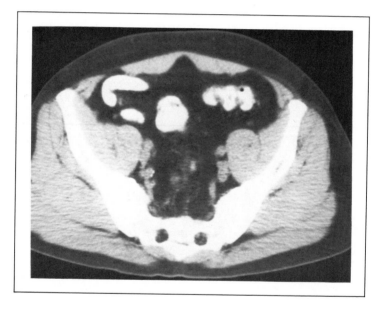

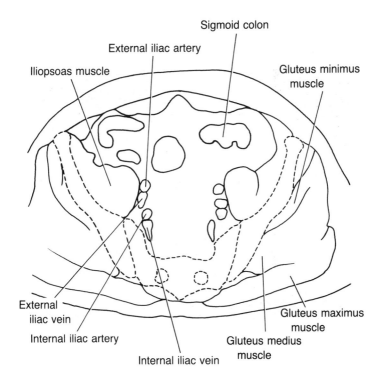

Sigmoid colon

External iliac artery

Iliopsoas muscle

Gluteus minimus
muscle

External
iliac vein

Internal iliac artery

Internal iliac vein

Gluteus maximus
muscle

Gluteus medius
muscle

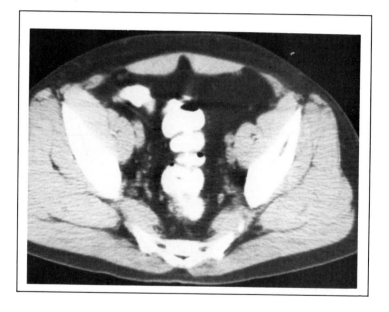

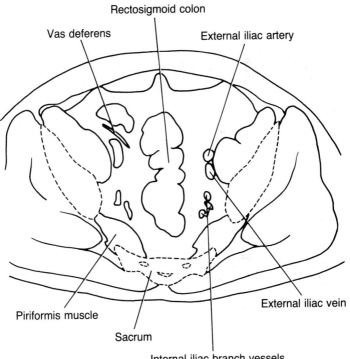

Rectosigmoid colon

Vas deferens

External iliac artery

Piriformis muscle

Sacrum

Internal iliac branch vessels

External iliac vein

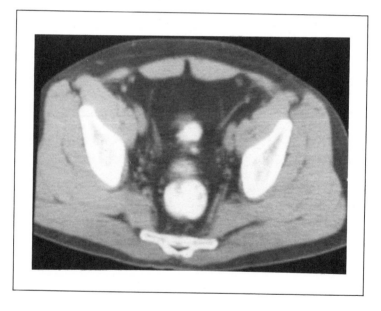

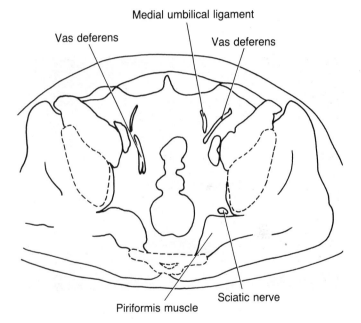

Medial umbilical ligament

Vas deferens

Vas deferens

Piriformis muscle

Sciatic nerve

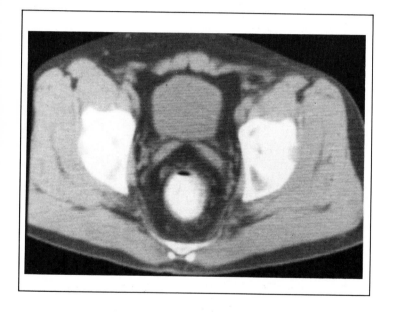

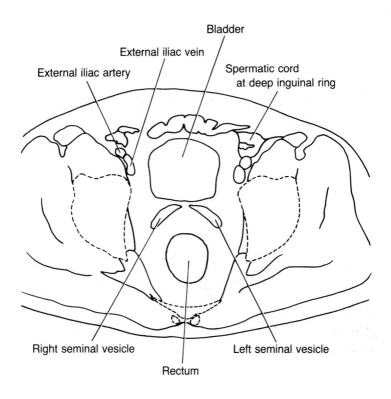

External iliac vein

Bladder

External iliac artery

Spermatic cord
at deep inguinal ring

Right seminal vesicle

Left seminal vesicle

Rectum

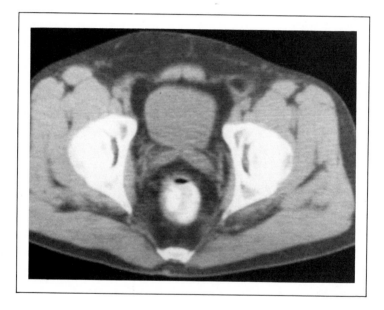

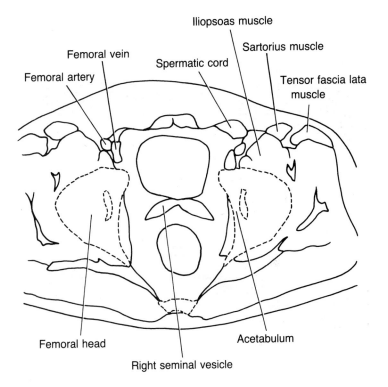

Iliopsoas muscle

Femoral vein

Sartorius muscle

Femoral artery

Spermatic cord

Tensor fascia lata
muscle

Femoral head

Acetabulum

Right seminal vesicle

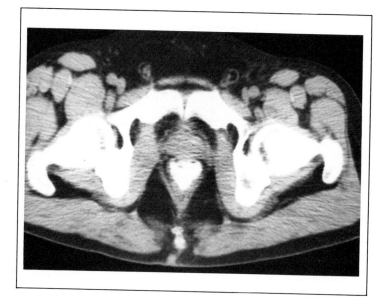

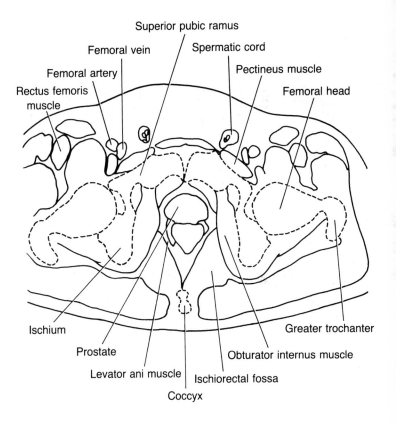

Superior pubic ramus

Femoral vein

Spermatic cord

Femoral artery

Pectineus muscle

Rectus femoris
muscle

Femoral head

Ischium

Greater trochanter

Prostate

Obturator internus muscle

Levator ani muscle

Ischiorectal fossa

Coccyx

Female Pelvis

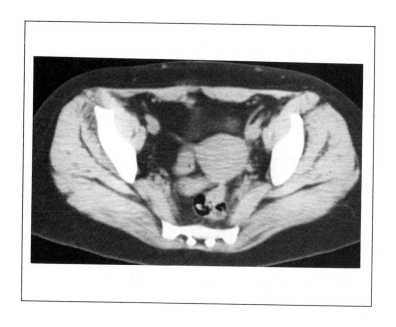

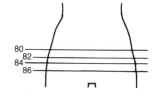

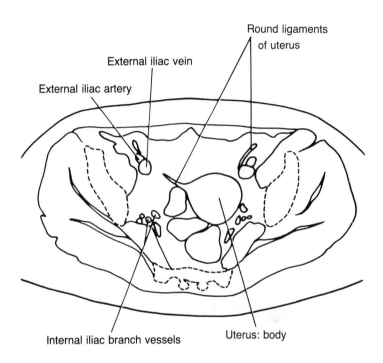

Round ligaments of uterus

External iliac vein

External iliac artery

Internal iliac branch vessels

Uterus: body

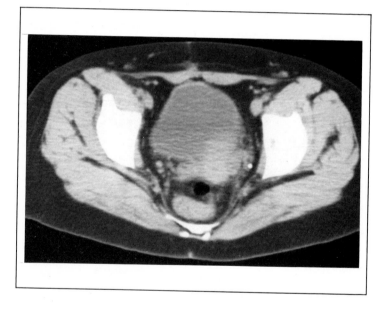

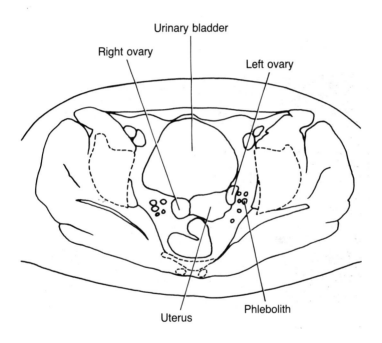

Urinary bladder

Right ovary

Left ovary

Uterus

Phlebolith

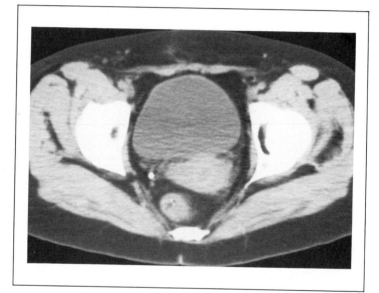

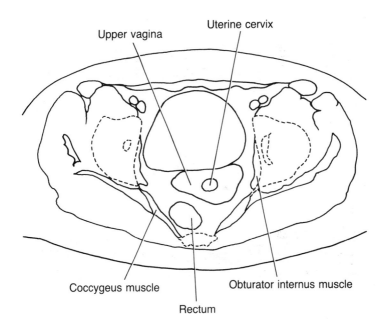

Upper vagina

Uterine cervix

Coccygeus muscle

Obturator internus muscle

Rectum

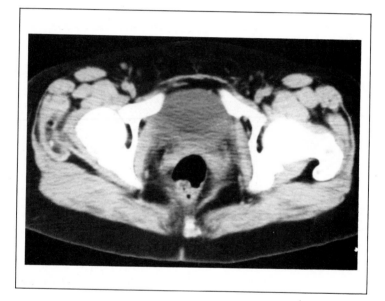

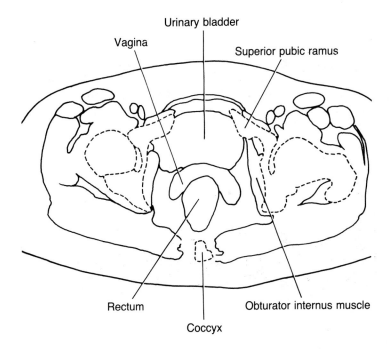

Urinary bladder

Vagina

Superior pubic ramus

Rectum

Obturator internus muscle

Coccyx